Eating Intuitively in a Diet-Crazed World

Ron Kness

Published by:

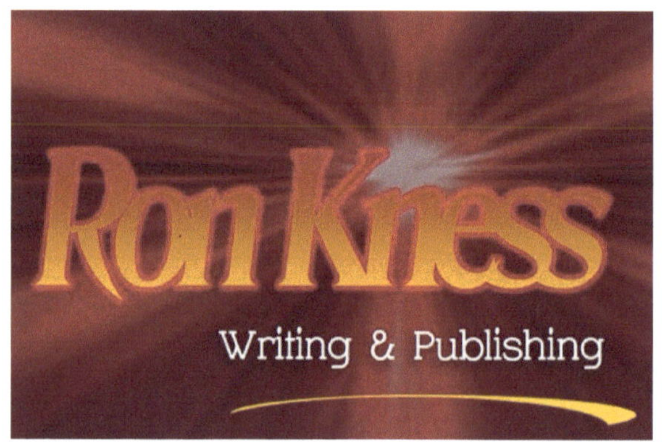

https://ronknesswriting.com

Ron Kness

Queen Creek, AZ

United States of America

ISBN: 9781708868420

Disclaimer

This eBook was written by Ron Kness. I am not a doctor or mental health professional and cannot be held liable for the information written here.

This book is meant to provide information about intuitive eating. For medical assistance, please seek help from a medical or mental health professional.

This publication is for informational purposes only and is not intended as medical advice. Medical advice should always be obtained from a qualified medical professional for any health conditions or symptoms associated with them.

Every possible effort has been made in preparing and researching this material. We make no warranties with respect to the accuracy, applicability of its contents or any omissions.

See your healthcare professional before starting any diet, health or exercise program!

Sneak Peek

People are often under the misconception that intuitive eating is just perpetuating obesity and unhealthy lifestyles, and just causing people to eat nothing but Oreo cookies and McDonald's fare. While it is true that many people eat foods they previously thought of as off-limits, they also eat a lot of nourishing food as well.

Intuitive eating is not a free-for-all where you eat whatever you want, in whatever quantity, regardless of how it makes you feel. It is all about honoring your hunger, trusting your body, and eating to fuel and nourish your body.

Here are some ways that intuitive eating works and can help you be the healthiest you have ever been.

It Relieves Stress About Food and Diets

To start with, you can relieve a lot of stress and frustration in your life when you begin intuitive eating. Think about how much time you spend thinking about food, researching diets, trying to plan your life around healthy meals, and the stress that comes from fear of hunger, binge and restrict cycles, and an obsession with how you look.

SO much of this is alleviated when you begin eating intuitively. All you must do is follow your body's cues, whether it means you are craving a juicy steak, or you are feeling like eating a big salad.

You Stop Obsessing About Food

You will also have a lot more free time when you aren't thinking about food. Intuitive eating helps you stop obsessing about every single thing you consume. Food just becomes food – that's all. It becomes a way to fuel your body, to nourish it with nutrients, to feel satisfied and happy. When you get to this point, you start noticing when you are actually hungry and when you are full, along with discovering the foods you love.

You Avoid Binge Cycles

This is a big deal for chronic dieters, people with disordered eating and eating disorders, and anyone who feels out of control around food. If you fear food, are afraid of sugar and fat, and think carbs are coming for you, then intuitive eating is the best option for you. In the beginning, it can be scary, but if you follow through with it, you will start to notice when you stop binging, and are able to just eat and not worry about it.

You No Longer Have Intense Cravings
Feel like you will always crave chocolate chip cookies or salty snacks forever? First of all, there is nothing wrong with these foods. Second, you will notice that you don't experience these intense cravings that seem to consume your mind. When you do have a craving, you will eat that thing to satisfy it, then move on. But you also understand when a craving is physical, or if it is an emotional pull from a history of restrictions. That is the beauty of intuitive eating.

Intuitive eating is a concept like no other you have tried. And unlike diets, which were only meant to be temporary, it is a healthy eating lifestyle you can live with for the rest of your life.

Before starting on your *Eating Intuitively in a Diet-Crazed World* journey, we suggest getting our companion 90-day journal/planner where you document your experience switching to this healthy eating lifestyle.

Why 90 days? Because it can take that long to get this new way of eating to become an instilled habit. You can purchase it at: https://www.amazon.com/dp/1707939969.

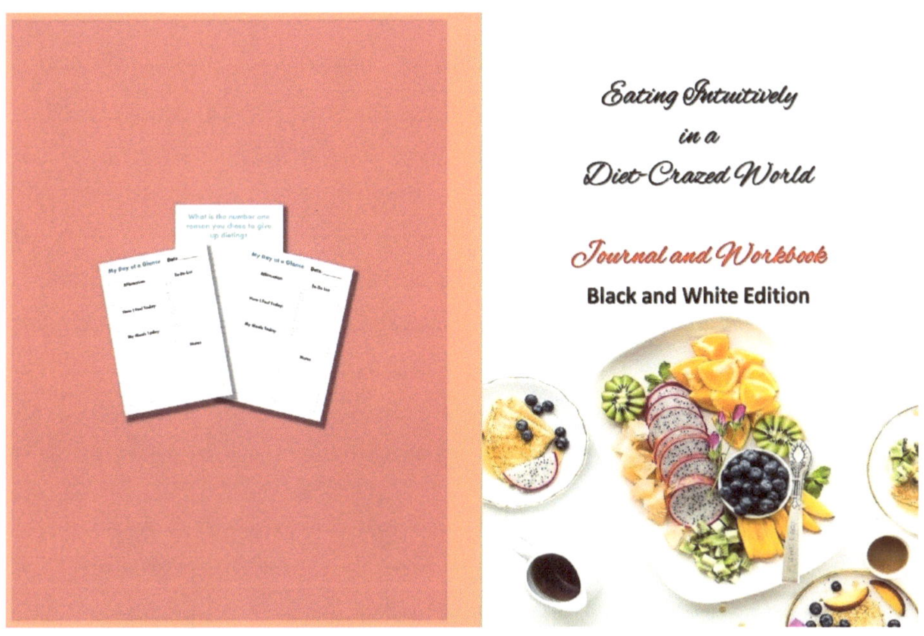

Table of Contents

Introduction

Intuitive eating is a way to change your lifestyle where you give up dieting for good, change your mindset about food and weight, and focus on living a healthier, more balanced life.

It is a hard transition to make in the beginning, since you completely remove your focus on your body and losing weight or getting #bodygoals, and instead focus on your mental health, and healing your relationship with food.

When you eat intuitively, to put it simple – you eat when you are hungry and stop when you are full. That is the basis of intuitive eating, but for people who have spent years of their life consumed by diet culture and food restrictions, it feels almost impossible.

This is how "normal eaters" eat, but if you have any sort of food restrictions in your past, whether actual dieting or just mental restrictions, learning about intuitive eating is the first step.

This book is going to guide you through some of the basic principle and methods introduced by the authors of the **Intuitive Eating Book**, Elyse Resche and Evelyn Tribole.

Throughout this book, you will learn:

- How to make peace with food.
- Learn how to trust your body.
- Nourish and fuel your body with any foods you want.
- Give up dieting forever.
- Make peace with your body and its signals.

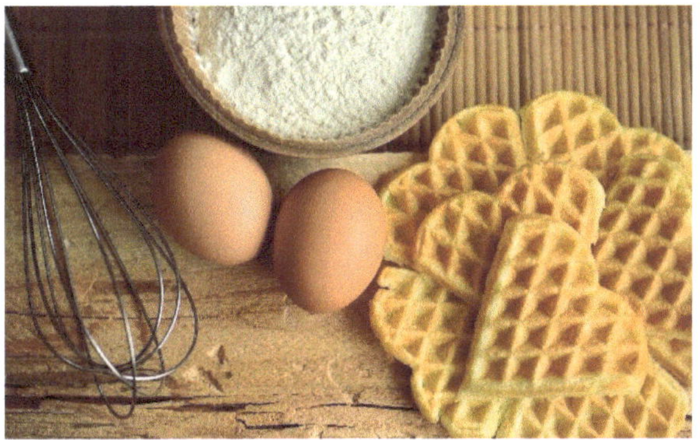

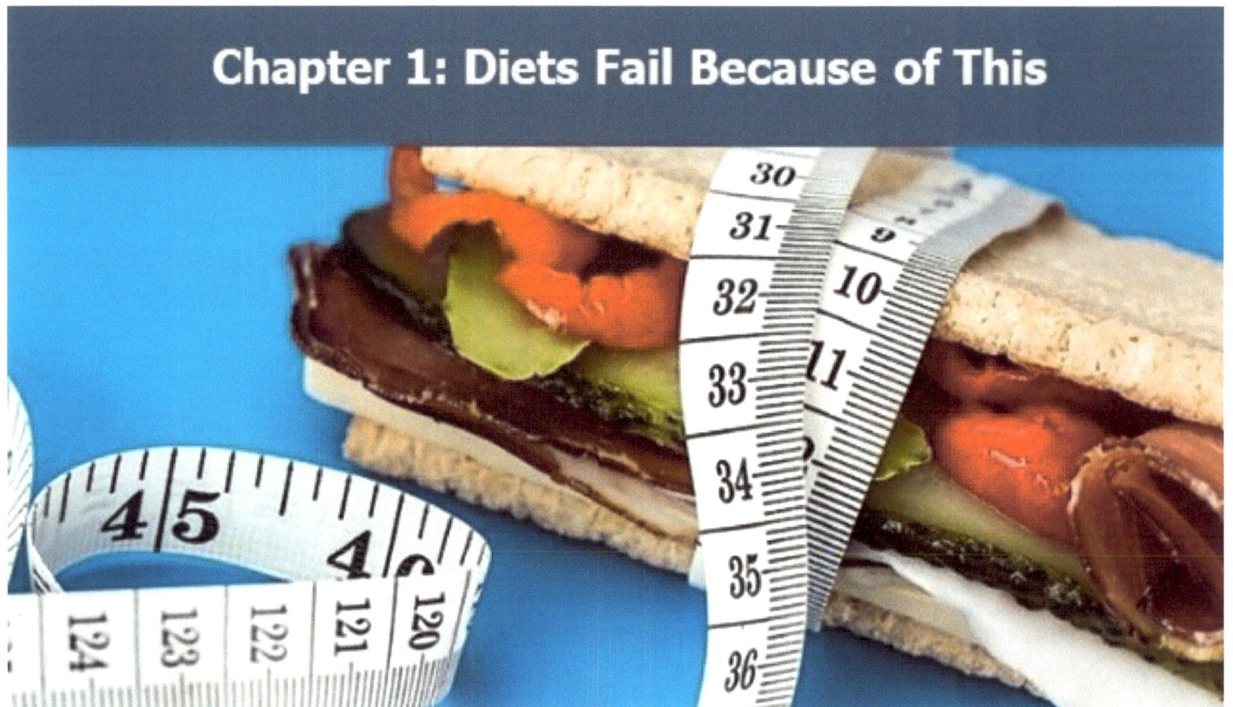

Chapter 1: Diets Fail Because of This

Diets are temporary. Let that sink in. *Diets are temporary.* They are not going to last forever. Not the diet, and rarely the results. The reason the statistics are so startling is because of all the promises diets give you. They promise to change your life, to make you happier, to make you healthier. They promise fast results, but they rarely promise you a lifetime of those results.

Why? Because companies that sell diet programs, pills, coaching programs, shakes, and food know that the long-lasting results are extremely rare.

Up to 95 percent of diets fail in the long-term. It is hard for people to accept because they have spent their lives wanting that dream body, to reach their "goal weight" and achieve what they have been promised.

You tell yourself that with enough willpower, enough endurance, and enough hard work, you can get there. As long as you stick to the plan, you will lose the weight and keep it off, and finally be happy. But remember what I said earlier … diets are temporary and so will be your results.

But what if you're not? What if you lose the weight and it comes back? What if you are like most people who spends your entire life bouncing from one diet to another, and never really find something you can stick to long-term?

What if the reason for that is because all diets fail... eventually. *What if that makes you normal?*

This chapter is going to cover the main reasons why diets fail, and why you are only setting yourself up for failure every time you jump back on a new diet bandwagon. And it shows you the importance of switching to an intuitive eating lifestyle. An eating lifestyle is something that you can live with forever … unlike diets that are temporary.

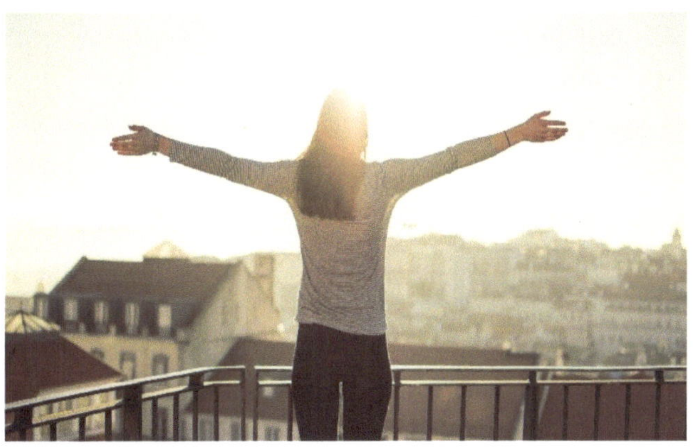

Diets are Not Meant for Long-Term Lifestyle Changes

According to countless studies, including the study performed at UCLA, the main reason dieting doesn't work, is because it doesn't last. This study found that while the participants lost 5-10 percent of their weight, the majority of them put it back on once off the diet.

Diets, at their core, are meant for short-term use only. Every diet out there "works" – until it doesn't. Sure, you might lose weight, mostly water weight in the beginning. If you stick with it, you might even lose fat. But most people find their way back to their old ways. They begin not only eating the foods they were restricting but overeating and binge eating them.

We will talk about this more in the next chapter, but this starts the inevitable binge-restrict cycle that people find so difficult to get out of.

If you want a quick fix that will only last until you start eating normally again, then by all means, keep dieting. But the sooner you realize it isn't working out for you and that there is a better way to live your life, the better off you will be.

Restriction Leads to Binges Which Lead to More Restrictions

Another reason diet fail for most people is because it can trigger the binge-restriction cycle. This is when you restrict in one way or another during your diet, then reach a point where you can't handle the restrictions, and suddenly "binge" on all the foods you were denying yourself. As you probably know, the cravings will win out every time!

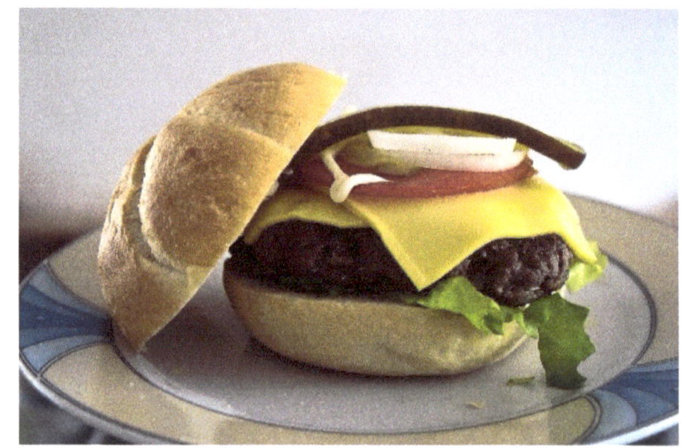

It is no surprise the foods you tend to binge on most often are the ones that you were not allowed to eat, or the foods you had guilt overeating. Maybe you were calorie counting and allowed yourself to eat anything within your calories – that doesn't mean you were mentally restricting. Telling yourself you shouldn't be eating that ice cream, because fruit would be much fewer calories and dairy-free and have less sugar.

This is the cycle you get into when you diet. Suddenly, food becomes nothing more than a number. You give it a moral value – good or bad. And eventually, most people will come back to those foods they were denying themselves, and more often than not, consume much more of them than they would have if they never restricted in the first place.

You Lose All Sense of Your Hunger and Fullness Cues

When you are on a diet, you are going based on numbers like calories and macros, meal timing, and the types of foods you are allowed to eat. What this does is keep you from actually gauging when you are hungry or full. You stop eating when the food you measured or weighed is done, not when you are full. Hungry between meals? *Oh well.* You must wait until the next meal, since your diet dictates what and when to eat.

This is one of many reasons why the hunger and fullness scale in the Intuitive Eating book is so helpful. It doesn't need to become something you perfect – but more of a way to start re-learning your own body's cues for how hungry you are, but also how full you are.

Eating Intuitively in a Diet-Crazed World

Believe it or not, if you come from a history of dieting and restricting, you probably don't even know how to tell when you are truly physically hungry, or how to stop eating when you're full. You eat within your allowed macros, and that's it.

There is so much more to eating for health and for fuel.

There are More Serious Risks …

In addition to the main reasons diets fail for many people, the National Eating Disorders Association found that dieting is actually one of the biggest risk factors for getting an eating disorder. Eating disorders like anorexia, bulimia, and the newly diagnosed binge eating disorder, can have dramatic and severe side effects on your health.

This is a very short list of the side effects people can experience from eating disorders:

- Digestive issues
- Gastrointestinal issues
- Nausea and vomiting
- Dehydration
- Malnutrition
- Low white blood cell count
- Increased risk of heart attack or stroke
- Mental health issues

The list goes on and on. And yes, people have died from their eating disorder, because of the health consequences.

Also, remember that you don't have to look emaciated to have an eating disorder. It comes in many forms, and people of all sizes can be suffering from an eating disorder.

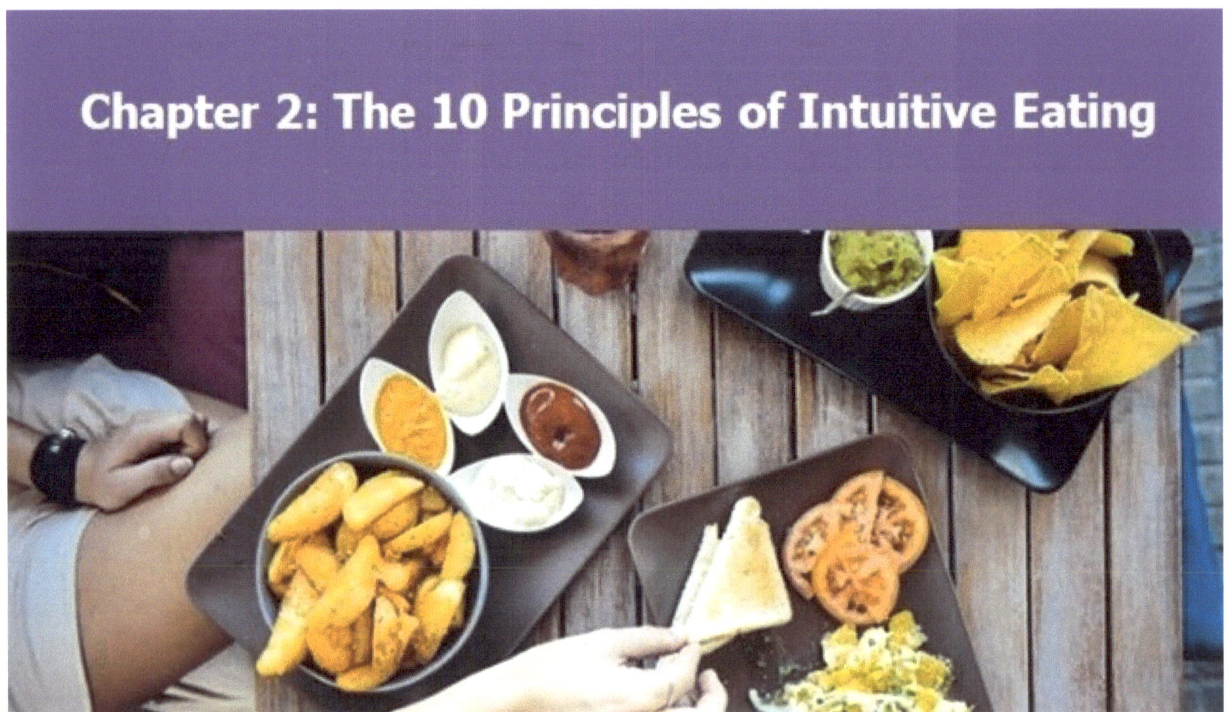

Chapter 2: The 10 Principles of Intuitive Eating

Now that you understand why diets fail and why you should be eating intuitively, let's go over some of the basics of what that means.

When you eat intuitively, you become a "normal eater". Everyone has those friends or family members who never seem to obsess about food. They don't think about food until they start getting hungry, they know when they are full, and they just go about their day once a meal is over.

This is the goal everyone wants to achieve, but for many people – a new diet is just around the corner. There are a lot of reasons for that, which may change based on your background, your body image, and the people you are surrounded by on a regular basis.

But what doesn't change is what you go through when you start intuitive eating. Elyse Resch and Evelyn Tribole wrote the original ***Intuitive Eating*** book, which came out originally in 1995, but has since gone through many updates to become what it is today.

This chapter is going to give you some insight into their original 10 Intuitive Eating Principles, with some notes and tips on each one so you know what to expect during each stage.

Principle 1: Reject the Diet Mentality

The first principle of Intuitive Eating, as mentioned in the book by Elyse Resch and Evelyn Tribole, is to reject the diet mentality. What does this mean? It is all about shutting down the diets, trying to steer clear of diet talk, and making a commitment to yourself that you will never diet or restrict again.

This is also a good place to remember that intuitive eating doesn't mean you will spend the rest of your life avoiding proper nutrition and nourishment, and instead just eat as much pizza, cereal, candy, and chips as you can get your hands on.

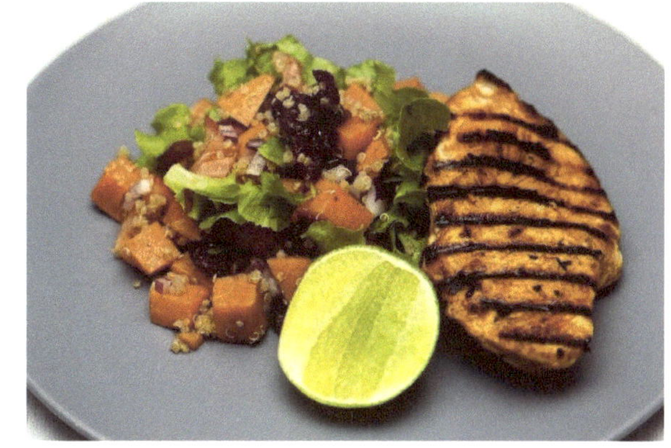

These foods are allowed, but so are whole grains, fruits, vegetables, breads, pastas and rice, seafood, meats of all kinds, and anything else your body wants and that sounds good to you.

However, you want to start your intuitive eating journey by saying no to diets. Delete those dieting and weight tracker apps from your phone, unfollow people who talk about diets on YouTube and Facebook and Instagram, throw away all the diet books and diet food in your house. If your scale is too tempting, get rid of that too!

You don't need these things anymore. They are no longer a part of your life. You are now committing to a life filled with good food that nourishes your body and gives you proper fuel and makes you happy and satiated. The restrictions are over.

Principle 2: Honor Your Hunger

With the Honor Your Hunger principle, you enter the honeymoon phase, sometimes called "all in" or "refeed". This is near the beginning of your intuitive eating and anti-diet journey, where you start eating when you are hungry, eat to satiation, and no longer restrict anything. And yes, that includes fried foods, dairy, gluten, grains, sugar, and whatever else you have been telling yourself you can't have.

During the Honor Your Hunger phase, you will eat whenever you feel hungry. In the beginning, it is going to feel like you are out of control, and like you will keep overeating forever. But everyone goes through these same fears, and they come out the other side understanding what their body wants and needs, and how to honor their hunger without feeling sick OR deprived.

You want to learn how to listen to your body's hunger and learn all about the hunger scale. The Intuitive Eating book shows you how to figure out how hungry or how full you are, which is going to help you on your journey. But during this phase, don't worry too much about the right amount of hunger or fullness. Just eat and refeed your body.

Principle 3: Make Peace with Food

Ready for Principle 3 of the Intuitive Eating book? This is when you are going to make peace with food. It often occurs at the same time as other principles and is definitely one of the most important things to remember.

Making peace with food means you are normalizing food, allowing all foods, and making sure you don't restrict anything. Pasta is no longer a "bad carb" – it's just pasta. Rice is just a grain, cheese is just a form of dairy, meat and seafood are just meat and seafood.

Remove the good and bad labels from your food and give yourself unconditional permission to eat anything you want. Do you want a bagel for breakfast? Great, have it! Are you thinking more about eggs? Make eggs! Are you in a hurry and only have time for a granola bar? Grab one and head out the door!

You don't need to try and rush this process, eating as much as you can in as little time as possible. Just slowly start thinking about food as fuel and a way to provide nourishment to your body, and that's it. It isn't evil, it isn't the enemy, and it isn't out to get you. And it isn't something you turn to for comfort when emotionally stressed.

Principle 4: Challenge the Food Police

What you will discover pretty early on in this journey to getting food freedom back is that you have an inner food police constantly trying to shut it down. It wants to tell you to be careful what you eat and how much you eat. This is closely tied to the labels you have in food, but it can sneak up on you in some subtle ways.

Maybe you are at a restaurant and even though the BLT sounds good, you skip the fries and get a side salad because it's better for you, or you decide to just get grilled chicken on a salad instead of the burger you actually want because you had carbs for breakfast.

There is nothing wrong with veggies and salads – you will soon discover your cravings for veggies, fruits, proteins, and all the other foods. But when you know your head and your food police are telling you two completely different things, that is when it becomes a problem.

This principle is all about challenging the food police. Asking yourself why you do or don't want something to eat, without worrying about what the police is trying to tell you. Thinking about what will make you feel good, what sounds good, what you are interested in eating. That's it.

There is no reason to feel guilt or shame about feeding your body. That is what you are supposed to do. Humans need food, and a wide variety of food, without cutting out entire food groups. Shut up your inner food police telling you what to eat and how much. Stop feeling guilty!

Principle 5: Respect Your Fullness

Moving on to Principle 5 – Respecting Your Fullness. In this principle, you use the hunger and fullness scale even more if you are intuitive eating. The scale goes from being ravenously hungry to so full you feel ill, and everything in between. You want to maintain an average level of satiation, where you aren't super full or super stuffed, but no longer hungry either.

It does take some time to learn how your body tells you when you are full. One strategy the Intuitive Eating book teaches you is to take pauses throughout your meal. If you have trouble remembering to do this, eat about half of your meal, then stop, take a drink of water, and wait a couple minutes.

If after those minutes, the food still sounds appetizing to you, you are probably still hungry. But sometimes, you lose interest and forget about it completely; that is a sign that you are reaching your fullness for now.

Principle 6: Discover the Satisfaction Factor

Principle 6 is all about your satisfaction factor, and while it seems simple, it is actually very important. What happens with people when they spend a lot of time dieting, is not only do they experience a lack of proper hunger and fullness signals, but they no longer get pure satisfaction from their food.

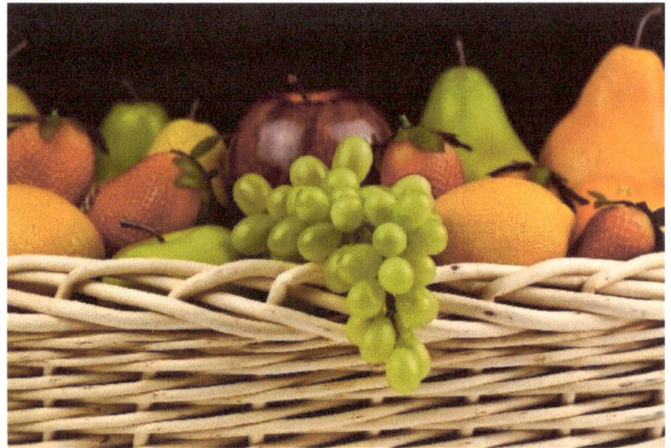

Maybe you are someone who eats while distracted, so you don't pay attention to what you're eating or how much, or you feel like you eat on autopilot without enjoying the tastes and sensations.

What this principle covers is teaching you how to find satisfaction, not only in the experience of eating, but in that feeling of being satiated and satisfied, without stuffed from overeating. It provides a good place to start with understanding when you are full.

And more importantly, you learn what it feels like to truly enjoy and be satisfied by your food. This is something that is almost impossible to attain when you are constantly on a diet.

Principle 7: Honor Your Feelings without Using Food

Time for Principle 7, where you are honoring your feelings without using food. Intuitive eating teaches you how to give up dieting, why health is subjective, and how to feel more freedom around food. But that doesn't mean you won't still experience things such as emotional or stress eating. While there is nothing inherently wrong with emotional eating, you want to learn other coping skills as well.

The main issue comes when food is the only coping mechanism you have. When no matter what you are going through, how you are feeling, or what struggles you have, you have absolutely nothing to help you find comfort other than food. That is when it can become a problem.

For this principle, intuitive eating teaches you how to honor your feelings, truly feel and experience them, and cope with them without using food to cover them up.

Principle 8: Respect Your Body

It is time to accept and respect your body for what it is, how it looks, and what it does for you. This part of intuitive eating is essential to giving up dieting for good. The majority of food issues don't start with food itself, but how we feel about our bodies. We live in a society where thinness is celebrated, and larger bodies are put down.

Where the size of your body is supposed to show how valuable you are, and if you are not in a publicly accepted body size, you are viewed as less than, unhealthy, lazy, and so many other untrue things.

While your body may change during the process of intuitive eating, including getting bigger OR smaller, that can't be the main focus. If your mind is still stuck on wanting to lose weight, you will never fully be able to find freedom around food, let go of your food guilt, and normalize food.

You need to stop criticizing your own body and letting what others think of you dictate what you should or shouldn't eat. This is one of the core principles of eating intuitively. It is important that you understand you cannot fully recover from binge eating or a toxic relationship with food and focus on weight loss at the same time. They just don't work together.

Principle 9: Exercise – Feel the Difference
Finally exercise becomes fun and healthy, not for weight loss! The second to last Intuitive Eating principle is about exercise. It is at the end of the list, because you really want to focus on food before you ever become active.

A general recommendation that many anti-diet dietitians give is to stop exercising until you feel ready to do so without thinking about it changing your body size or shape. Again, you want to focus on how exercise makes you feel, not how it can change what your body looks like.

You will learn how to exercise for health, for happiness, for energy, and for life – not for weight loss.

Principle 10: Honor Your Health

Lastly, this principle is about honoring your health. In the Intuitive Eating book, you will learn WHY this is the last principle. It is sometimes hard to separate health from weight loss or weight management, which is why it should be the very last thing you work on.

Honoring your health focuses on gentle nutrition. Not restricting certain foods, aiming for the perfect balance of nutrients every time, or making sure you don't "overeat". Instead, you are still going to follow your cravings and taste buds, and let your body guide you to your own version of nutrition.

It might look different for everyone. You want to fuel your body, nourish it with the good stuff, but never restrict anything unless you have a serious food allergy. There is a BIG difference between not eating bread because you are Celiac or have flare-ups from Crohn's disease, than not eating it because you think carbs will cause you to gain weight.

This is when you understand the difference.

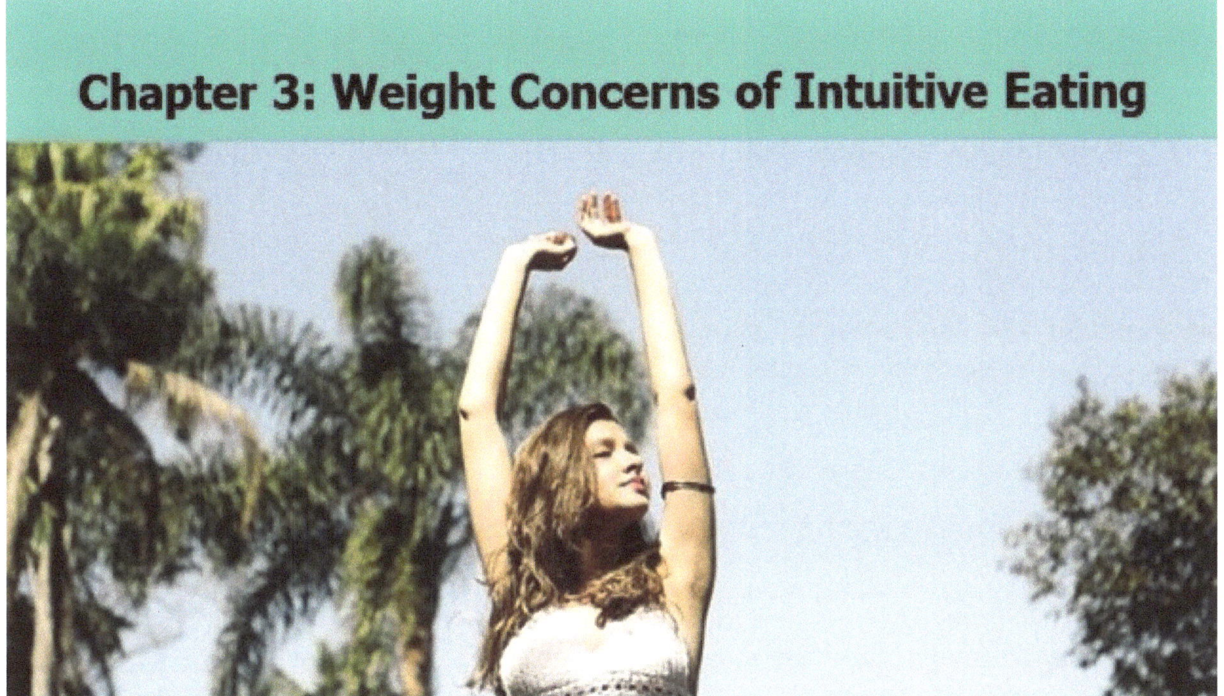

Chapter 3: Weight Concerns of Intuitive Eating

The big question of intuitive eating and one of the main reasons people are hesitant to ditch the diet mentality is the fear of weight gain.

Will you gain weight? Maybe.

There are no guarantees about what will happen to your body as you go through this process. You will learn through intuitive eating that you need to honor your hunger, trust your body, and put aside thoughts of how your body looks and the size of your body, and instead focus on healing your relationship with food.

If you are worried about weight gain and that is the reason why you don't want to try intuitive eating, ask yourself this question first:

Why are you so afraid of gaining weight?

Be honest with yourself. Are you worried about your health? Or is it more about what other people will think? If most of your concerns have to do with what other people will think or say, then it has nothing to do with YOU. This is your body and your life, and your choice about whether or not you are ready to fully commit to intuitive eating and heal your relationship with food once and for all.

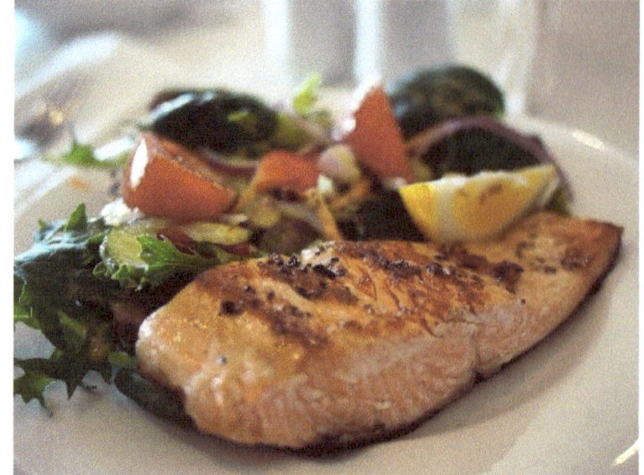

In this third chapter, we are going to talk all about weight concerns, including whether you might gain weight, and how to deal with it if you do.

Will You Gain Weight When You Start Eating Intuitively?

Unfortunately, nobody can answer this question for you. But the most important thing to remember is that with intuitive eating, you are no longer focusing on the size of your body or how much you weigh. Get rid of the scale and stop worrying about what your body is doing. Focus on how your body feels instead.

There is a lot that goes into weight loss and weight gain. It is much more complex than what you might think, and your body is going to do everything it can to get to the weight it wants to be at.

Who is More Likely to Gain Weight – While there is no telling what is going to happen to your weight, people are coming directly from a period of restricting their food and extreme exercise to intuitive eating are more likely to gain more weight, at a more rapid pace. Your body needs time to catch up to your new diet. It needs to learn to trust that it will keep being fed and won't face another period of restriction or starvation.

This extra weight is a good thing. Your body is going what it is meant to – holding onto extra weight just in case another famine is around the corner.

What to do When You Gain Weight – Don't panic! Weight gain is nothing to worry about. I know – easier said than done. Depending on your history with your weight and relationship with dieting, it may take you a while before you get used to the new shape and size of your body. But keep in mind weight fluctuates many times throughout your life, for many reasons. Food is not the enemy, and neither is a little fat on your bones.

Overshooting Your Set Weight – There is a lot of science when it comes to set weight theory, which you will learn in just about every intuitive eating and anti-diet book out there. But the summary is this: everyone has a set weight. This is the weight where your body feels most comfortable. You feel good, energized, and your body just works really great.

This does NOT mean you personally enjoy being at this weight unfortunately. It may be the last thing you want, it may be 20, 30, 50 pounds over your old goal weight. And it can be raised by overshooting, which usually is the result of binge eating or overeating.

If it helps, many people who overshoot their set weight during intuitive eating, when you start allowing all foods, will end up losing some of that weight and go back down to their normal set weight.

Can You Eat Intuitively if You Are Overweight?

Yes! Intuitive eating is for everyone. While a lot of people who do intuitive eating are coming from a background of severe restrictions and often eating disorders, that doesn't mean you have to be thin or have a history of binge eating for it to be successful for you.

Intuitive eating is the most basic form of eating. It is a way to get back to normal eating, the way you were born to eat. It doesn't matter who you are, the size of your body, your history with dieting, or how much you weigh – you can benefit from eating more intuitively.

It is still a good idea to talk to your doctor about potential medical conditions you are managing but remember even if you need to avoid certain foods because of a condition like diabetes or Celiac, doesn't mean you can't also be an intuitive eater.

Why You Can't Focus on Weight Loss and Intuitive Eating at the Same Time

Intuitive eating and weight loss work against each other. It is impossible to do one correctly, while also doing the other. You need to get to a point where you say goodbye to diets, and you accept your body for what it is and accept all the changes that may or may not come.

Try to imagine a scenario where you allow all foods, stop dieting and stop tracking, have no more food restrictions, and follow your cravings. Now picture yourself also trying to lose weight while doing that.

It doesn't work, right? That is because a big part of intuitive eating is letting go of those dreams of a certain body type, accepting your body as it is and as it was meant to be, and finding the food freedom you crave.

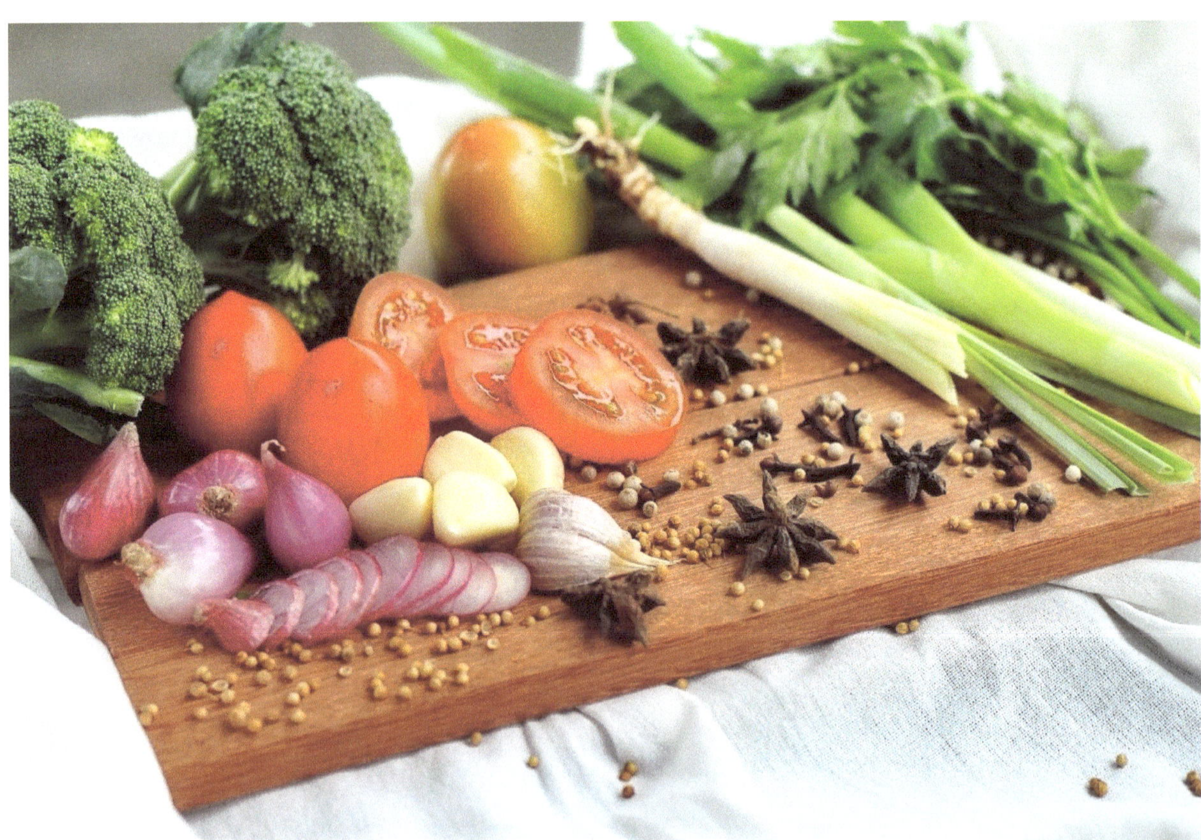

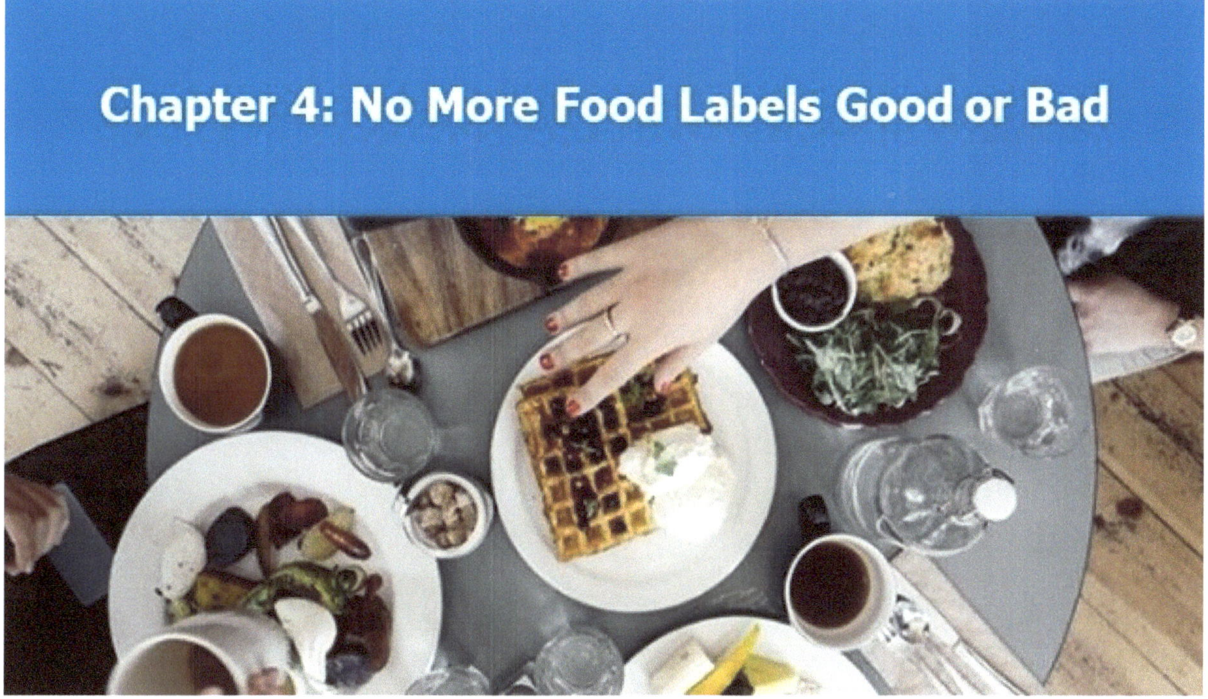

Chapter 4: No More Food Labels Good or Bad

The first three Intuitive Eating principles are all related to food, healing your relationship with food, and removing the "good" and "bad" labels you have from your food. This is often referred to as the honeymoon period, as it is when you allow ALL foods, no matter what they are, their ingredients, how they were made, what macronutrients they contain, and in what quantities you want to eat them.

This can be a scary process, but it is essential that you do this first before anything else, so that you can normalize food. You want to neutralize food, and remove all those numbers and labels. No food is good or bad, it's just food. It nourishes your body in different ways.

For this chapter, we really want you to understand the importance of removing the good and bad labels from your food, and how to learn how to listen to your body as you begin intuitive eating.

Food is Just Food

To remove those labels you have from food – including the ones you think about mentally, without considering them restrictions – you have to neutralize food. This doesn't mean you don't enjoy certain foods, but that you accept food for what it is: just food.

It is there to give you energy, fuel your body, keep you satiated, and keep you alive. And yes, it can help you feel better, cheer you up, help bring families together, and celebrate special occasions.

What it no longer does is make you feel shame or guilt, define how healthy or unhealthy of a person you are, dictate whether or not you are a person worthy of love and respect, and no longer has control over you.

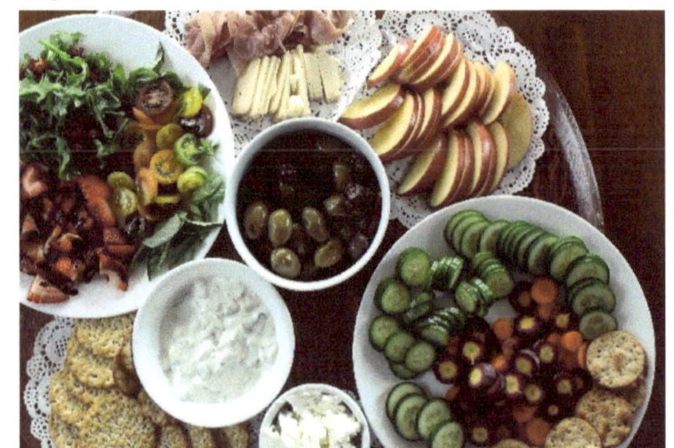

Food does not have a moral value. It is not good or bad, right or wrong. It isn't there to hurt you or punish you or reward you. Food is there to fuel you, give you energy, and FEED YOU! That's it. The sooner you can learn how to normalize your food, the easier it will be to keep living an intuitive eating lifestyle.

Do You Still Have Mental Food Restrictions?

One thing people struggle with is the mental food restrictions that you don't always notice you have. These can be small and subtle but affect you just as much as when you have actual dieting restrictions.

For example, if you still consider sugar to be bad for you, that is a restriction. Even if you still eat sugar, but you feel guilt for eating it or eating "too much" of it, that is still a restriction.

Still confused? Here are some common signs that you have mental food restrictions:

- You don't eat what you crave, because you think it's fattening, bad for you, or you already ate too much that day.
- You skip a meal purposely after eating a big meal.

- You mentally tell yourself no, you shouldn't, or you can't eat a certain thing.
- You increase workouts purposely on days where you feel like you ate too much.
- You feel intense guilt after eating certain types of foods or certain quantities.

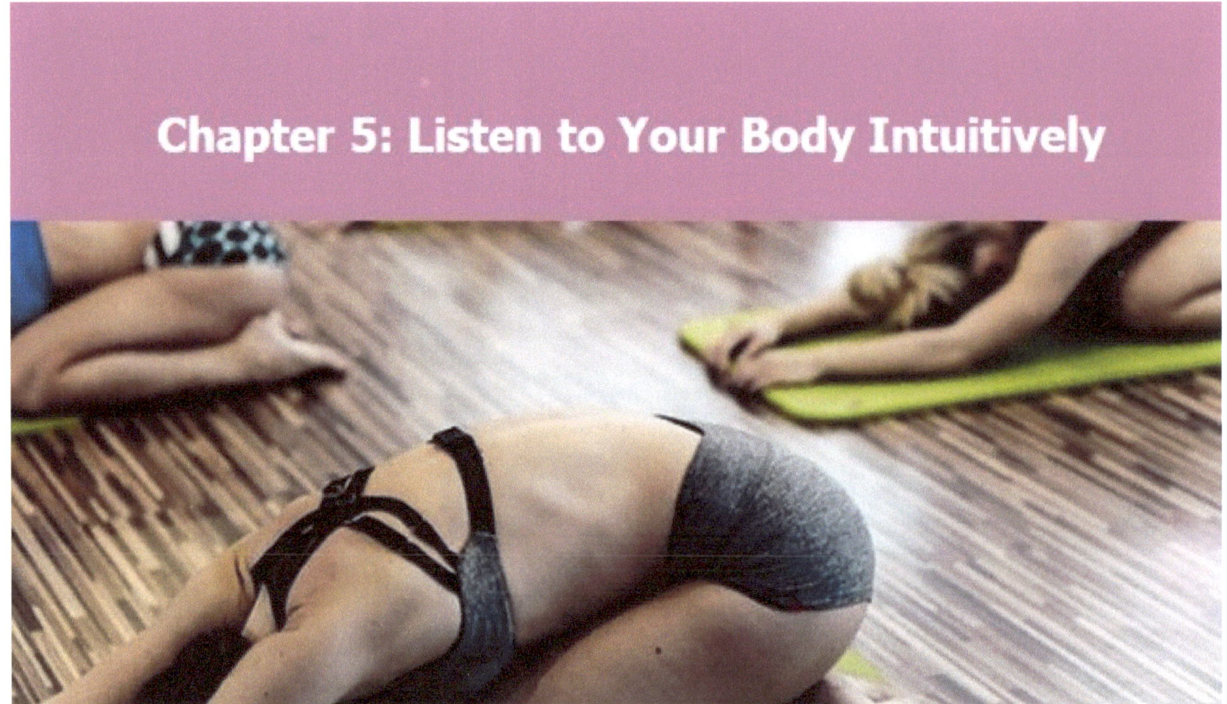

Chapter 5: Listen to Your Body Intuitively

When You Feel Out of Control

Do you still feel out of control with your food? If so, just be patient with yourself and take the intuitive eating process one step at a time.

In the beginning, when you are honoring your hunger and cravings, you are only focusing on allowing yourself to eat without criticism and without limits.

You are going to ask yourself if you are eating too much, whether or not this will ever stop, and if you are going to eat yourself into morbid obesity.

You aren't. This phase is very important. It can feel scary when you aren't controlling what you are eating and how much, but you will never be able to fully be an intuitive eating without first allowing all foods and making sure nothing is off limits.

It is common to assume healing your relationship with food is just about food, but it is so much more than that. You are also healing your relationship with yourself and with your own body.

You have likely spent a long time criticizing your body, hating it for its size, wishing it would change, and feeling anger or resentment over being hungry when you think you should be full, or craving foods you have put on your "bad' food list.

This all leads to a toxic relationship with yourself. It may have started with food, but it doesn't end there.

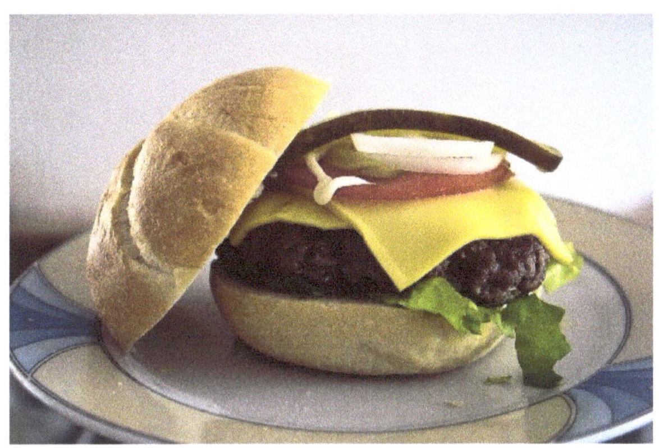

With intuitive eating, you need to learn how to listen to your body. You will learn how to know when you are hungry and when you are full, use your own version of the food scale, and understand what your body is trying to tell you.

The most important thing to remember is that it is not a linear process, nor a short one. You need to be patient with yourself and try to listen to the signs your body is telling you, but not stress too much about it.

Here are some tips for learning how to listen to your body as you begin on your intuitive eating journey.

Trusting Your Body

Whether you have spent a few years wanting to lose weight, or over a decade despising your body, it is time to trust it and let it end up where it is going to end up naturally.

Our bodies are very smart. They know what they're doing. We have set weight ranges each of our bodies wants to be at. It will work very hard against you to get there. This is why it seems like your weight is always about the same no matter how much or how little you eat after a certain point.

Why diets feel like they aren't working, and why sometimes when you eat MORE than you expected, you don't always gain weight.

Your body is trying to protect you. Stay at the weight it naturally wants to be at. When you go on extreme diets and force your body to get smaller, you are only setting yourself up for failure.

During the intuitive eating process, it takes a lot of trust. You are handing over control, and letting your body do what it is meant to do. This is very scary. But the more you can learn how to really trust in the process and understand that your body will end up wherever it ends up, the more food freedom you will have.

Hunger and Cravings

When you are respecting and trusting your body, you are also giving in to all your cravings and eating when you feel hungry. Over time, you will learn the difference between physical hunger and emotional hunger and be able to navigate this much more easily. But for now – just honor those cravings and feed yourself the proper nourishment when your body needs it.

It is as simple as this:

1. If you are hungry, eat. That's it. Eat when you feel hungry or feel like eating. The hunger signals vary person to person, so it may take some getting used to when you first become more in tune with your body.

2. If you crave something, satisfy that craving. The more you try to put off your cravings and avoid them purposely, the stronger they become. Before too long, you are eating an entire carton of ice cream, where you might have been satisfied with a bowl. Just eat what you are craving when it is available.

3. If you're still hungry after a meal, eat again. Yes really. Your body is telling you that it wasn't enough food to fuel up and to nourish your body. Your hunger will change day by day. This is normal and what is supposed to happen. If it's a day when your hormone levels are fluctuating or after you ate a smaller meal or when you worked out, you're going to be hungrier. Just follow your body's lead.

Mindfulness

While it isn't mandatory to eat intuitively, eating more mindfully is highly recommended. This is when you remove distractions and focus on what you are eating, how it tastes and smells, and how it makes you feel.

Mindfulness allows you to appreciate your food more and find that satisfaction factor you have been missing while dieting and feeling like food is there to hurt you.

How to Eat More Mindfully:

- Turn off all distractions – Try to eat at least one meal a day without any distractions. This means sitting at a table eating, without using the computer, listening to music, or watching podcasts.
- Chew slowly – Chew more slowly and succinctly. Not uncomfortably slow, but not rushing through your meal without even feeling satisfaction.
- Take breaks between bites – This is part of chewing slowly, but you also don't want to rush in between bites. Take breaks, put your fork down, and just sit quietly for a minute. This helps you remain mindful, but also gauge when you have reached your comfortable satiety level.
- Enjoy the sensations – Being more mindful about your food is like meditating. But instead of clearing your mind of everything, you clear your mind of everything but the food. Enjoy each sensation, including the flavor, texture, taste on your tongue, and how enjoyable the food is to you.

Gentle Nutrition

Finally, there is a place for focusing on nutrition in intuitive eating, even though in the beginning it can feel like all you are eating is pizza and chocolate chip cookies. This is called a "honeymoon period" for a reason – it doesn't last forever.

What does gentle nutrition mean?

Focusing on nutrition is often combined with dieting and restrictions (even subtle restrictions), so the authors of Intuitive Eating added a 10th principle that is often nicknamed gentle nutrition.

It is to help you understand that not only is intuitive not just about eating cookies and chips for the rest of your life and that nutrition is still important, but that you want to do it in a healthy, balanced, non-diet way.

Then the concept of gentle nutrition was born. It is all about balance, and eating a wide range of foods. You want to eat what you enjoy, what fuels your body, and what feels good, without ever depriving yourself.

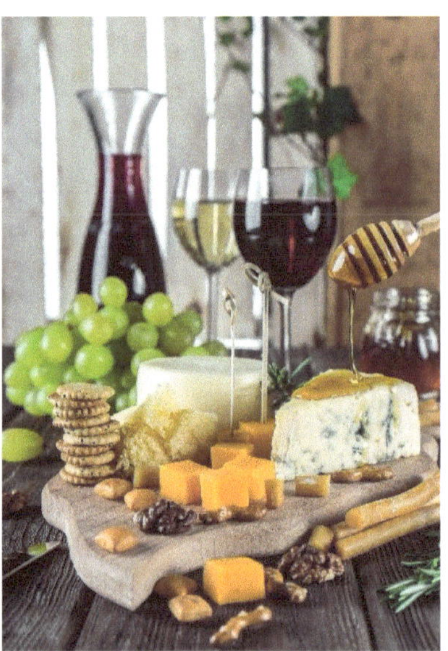

Tips for Adding Gentle Nutrition into Your Life

1. Get a balance of nutrients, without rules. In the past, if you have tried to "give up dieting" and instead "eat a balanced diet" it probably still consisted of some rules. Like always combining protein, fat, and carbs, or making sure you had veggies with every meal. While there is nothing wrong with this, some people turned it into another set of food rules.

The point of intuitive eating is to just eat, nourish your body, and STOP dieting. Giving up ALL food rules. That means balance is going to be different. Some days, you eat salmon, rice, and veggies for dinner because it sounds good. Other days, you eat a side salad with your burger, or you go for the fries with your burger.

There are so many ways to get essential nutrients from your food, and it isn't going to look the same every meal, or every day.

2. Pay attention to what feels good. As you progress further with intuitive eating, you will have a mental tally of foods that make you feel good, and foods that make you feel not so good. Maybe some foods sap your energy, so instead of eating them earlier in the day, you save them for the nighttime when you're relaxing.

Or you have found certain types of foods are delicious but hurt your tummy a little. While other meals are absolutely perfect, and really just make you feel so good and energized.

These are things to pay attention to when you start incorporating gentle nutrition.

3. Be as loose as you can with your meals. This means not paying so much attention to the right foods at the right time or timing your meals perfectly. Of course, if you have lunch breaks at certain times, that is when you will eat lunch, but don't feel like you are forced to eat a certain meal at a specific time during the day.

Be loose with your meals, where you just eat when you're hungry, eat what sounds good at the time, then move on with your life. This is what intuitive eating is – fueling your body and getting that diet voice out of your head.

Final Thoughts

Intuitive eating is for everyone. Don't worry if you don't feel like you have restricted enough or you don't have disordered eating. If you are reading about eating more intuitively, you probably have some type of toxic relationship with food that you want to change.

It looks different for everyone. Don't put too much pressure on yourself to change all your ways overnight, feel like you're not doing it correctly, or that it isn't working.

Be kind to yourself and kind to your body. It's not a linear process, but it is so worth it.

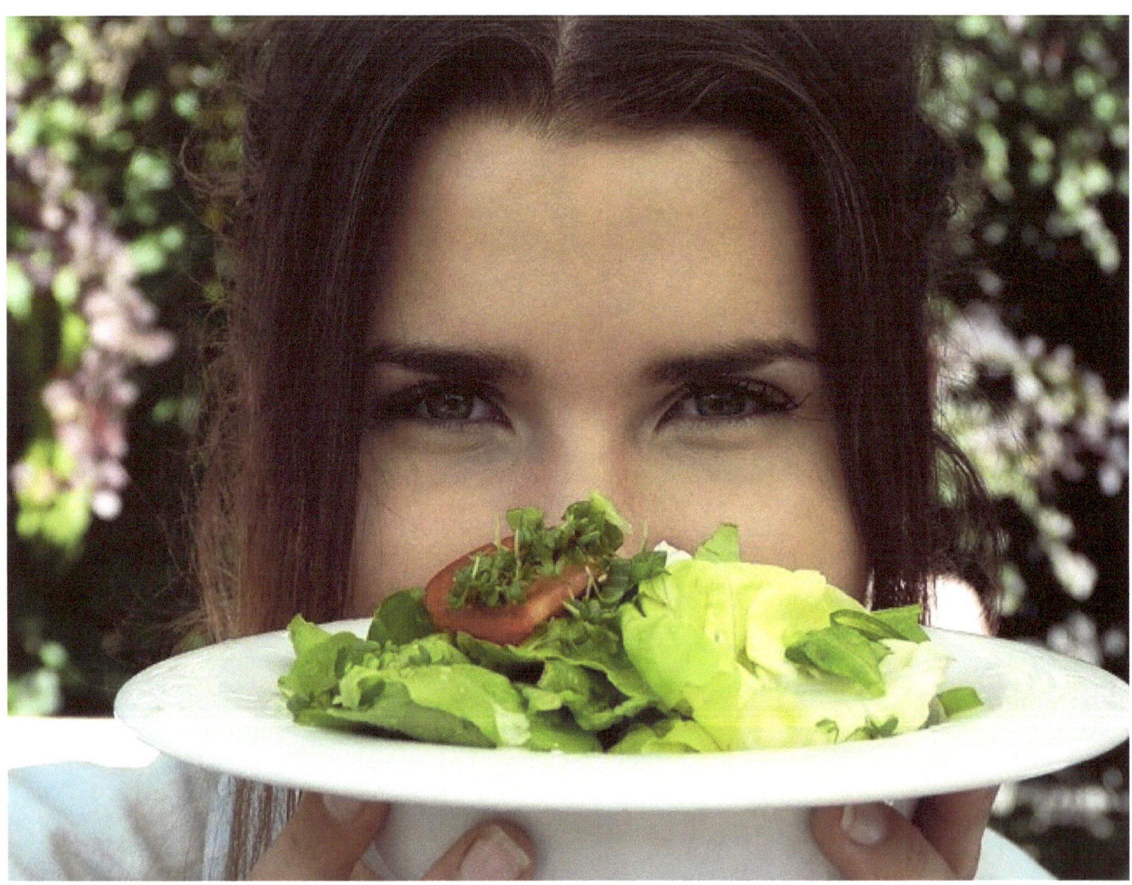

About the Author

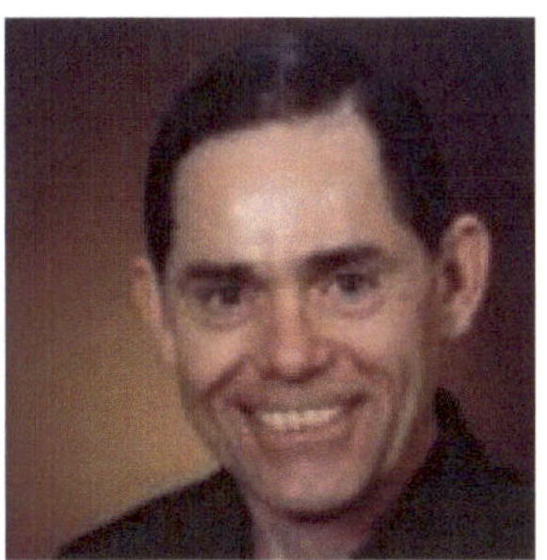

I have published numerous books on Amazon (both for Kindle and in paperback), along with other publishing platforms.

While most of my books are on health and fitness in general, I also write on baby boomer and older citizen health issues and have a recent interest in creating and printing journals/ planners and other printable products.

Besides my own writing, I also ghostwrite ebooks, books, reports, articles, blogs and do Kindle conversions for clients on a variety of topics.

Go to my website at http://ronknesswriting.com for more information or to submit a quote. For a complete list of my books, go to https://www.amazon.com/Ron-Kness/e/B0072M6PYO.

Today my wife and I are retired from our careers and live in Queen Creek, AZ. I now write as a retirement business where you'll find me happily sitting in my office typing away on my laptop as I work on my next book or ghostwriting project . . . that is if we are not traveling on a cruise ship - our new-found mode of travel.